Stress

MW00804282

Effective Ways of Reducing Stress & Boosting Immune System Naturally with Self-Help That Works for Kids and Adults

Emily Melanie

Copyright © 2020

All rights reserved. No part of this publication may be reproduced, distributed, or transmitted in any form or by any means, including photocopying, recording, or other electronic or mechanical methods, without the prior written permission of the publisher, except in the case of brief quotations embodied in critical reviews and specific other non-commercial uses permitted by copyright law.

Table of Contents

Introduction

Are you aware that managing your stress is as important as keeping a constant watch on your health?

Do you know the effects of properly managed stress on your immune system building capability?

This book will take you through the steps you need to follow to effectively manage your stress and also that of your children's the natural way

You will find several ways to manage stress, such as controlling your thoughts, managing your emotions, eating healthy, exercising regularly, and more. This book also gives information about how to detect stress in kids, the symptoms, stress-relieving games that would help both kids and adults, stress-relieving exercises, what makes children anxious and what parents are expected to do, and how positive thinking can assist you in healing and ultimately move forward in life.

People who figure out how to deal with stress and business live a happier and healthier life because a sound body is a formidable tool to fight stress.

As you read further on what to do to help your children manage stress effectively and also to manage your own stress. You would be glad you did because this book explains basic mechanisms of stress and relaxation and offers research-based guidance for improving treatment outcomes.

Chapter 1

Identifying Stress in Kids

Through the bogeyman for young kids towards the bogies of SATs as well as the last exams designed for the college-bound, it's been carefully observed that stress affects children of all ages; one thing a father or mother can do to significantly help a youngster manage anxiety and stress is to make a significant family decision, which includes constant conversation with the youngster to get familiar with his/her psychological state to be tensed.

Children, especially those with under-developed communications abilities, may experience screen anxiety in different ways compared to grown-ups. Often time, children's stress is usually internalized and, most apparently, in a physically perceived sensation for example regular flu-like symptoms, such as headache, stomachache, as well as nausea.

Children below anxiety might regress to habits like bedwetting, clinginess, and regular crying; these symptoms may be intense, as an ordinarily energetic child turns into either listless or hyper-active, a generally docile kid has suits of anger or a youngster that "functions out" becomes bright and reflective.

Some indications of stress in children are often confused with children's mental disorders. For instance, your child's good friend goes through an extreme switch, anxiety, and emotional stress might be part of it at this time, for example, that may reveal a child's inability to deal with the demanding circumstance.

As much as stress can be an integral part of grown-ups' lives today, so it is progressively a vital feature of kids' lives as well, this implies that stress administration for kids ought to be an initial topic parent must comprehend and understand. Child stress and matured stress often occur due to several factors which may be entirely resolved by merely studying the actual problem resulting in child stress, and going through the process of helping a youngster become better and calmer.

Chapter 2

Factors behind Stress

Stress could be thought to have one cause, which may be the awareness and response towards the conditions that happen inside our lives. Stress could be triggered by just something as easy as breaking a fingernail. Also, the positive events in our lives tend to be as nerve-racking as the harmful ones.

For example, the delivery of a youngster could be stressful, negatively and positively. If the infant is a boy or a girl, no matter how beautiful the child is at that moment, our adrenaline moves and down with satisfaction since our minds fill up with jubilation and overwhelming feelings. Frequent stress allows numerous thoughts to begin to run through your head, e.g., "Am I going to be a good father or mother? "Will I be able to have other babies? Am I going to have to wake up at 2am every morning to tend my crying child?"

There are two basic types of stress, the first; Eustress or

Positive pressure, and the latter is Distress or Unfavorable anxiety. Coping with stress is more straightforward than dealing with pain; the fact remains that stress can either be positive or negative.

Furthermore, what would relieve someone else's stress might stress another person out. For instance, "Divorce could be seen as alleviation for one party" or "a calamity that leads to loss of job, which may provide one with an essential holiday and at the same time could result in financial upheaval."

Whatever stresses people out or causes stress is called a Stressor. Usually, the sort of stress many people are concerned about is "Distress", a processive stressor or systemic stressors can trigger this negative stress.

Processive stressors generate what's referred to as the "fight or flight" reaction. If we believe there's a severe immediate danger, the pituitary gland instantly noises a burglar alarm by merely liberating a burst of adrenocorticotropic body hormone (ACTH), which indicates the adrenal glands and releases the "human stress hormones" that is adrenaline and cortisol.

These human hormones are actually glands that help us focus on the situation, increase response timing, and briefly increase our physical power and agility while we determine whether to retreat or stand.

A systemic stressor may be the body's automated physiological reactions to stress, just like the insufficient equilibrium (dizziness) that you feel before you faint or possibly the discharge of acid solution that turns and churns your stomach in a nerve-racking scenario.

The systemic stressor could be released concurrently along with processive stressors and could cause a lot more stress because they pose a lot of risk to your overall health.

Although everyone has at one time or the other undergone stress, study indicates that children who grow up in burdensome areas are in higher threat of being apprehensive by life's challenges.

Furthermore, some analysis experimented in both progressive and systematic occasions. People find the ability to handle the tension triggered by these occasions, partially due to hereditary, governed by genes that control the endorphin amounts. (Endorphins would be the human hormones that control the moods and also become an all-natural "pain killer").

Although events might appear stress filled, it's necessary to take into account that stress is produced by our reactions to circumstances.

The simple truth is stress could be "all inside our mind." Placing life's fluctuations into proper perspective may be the first approach to coping with anxiety, and the result is usually seen in our lives and well-being.

Chapter 3

Symptoms of stress

The symptoms of anxiety are our physical, psychological, and behavioral responses to life's situations.

·   The pounding of our hearts as the home team reaches the winning point.

·   The sensation of disappointment when the other team scores a goal.

·   The wild jubilation when we win as well as the anger we feel when we lose out.

Examples of stress are classified as Extreme, Episodic Severe, and Persistent. Stress symptoms tend to be considered a sign of the amount of anxiety. Severe anxiety may be the short-term sort of pressure we experience, for instance, if we stand back on the curb away from the oncoming vehicle, or when the home team wins (or loses).

This type of stress may be the most workable. Our center rates leap, bloodstream stresses raise, pressure headaches might ensue, most of us become briefly upset, optimistic, boisterous, or resentful. Most of us cry in pleasure, in comfort, or even in frustration.

Episodic severe stress occurs when life's situations happen to people. Among these is when life's situation rotates uncontrollably with one devastation upon another - a sickness, a divorce, and unfinished work in some time.

Symptoms like recurring headaches, indigestion, exhaustion, and sleep problems are vibrant indicators of Episodic desperate stress. We can prevent occasional severe stress by realizing its signs and coping with difficult circumstances because they happen. Without this, the amount of stress can lead to chronic anxiety.

Chronic anxiety/stress is whatever stresses one out, grinding one down till our bodies and minds respond with severe long-term physical or mental disorders. Persistent tension occurs when circumstances become challenging to handle when there's "no way out," and we quit wanting to conquer adversity.

Regrettably, once stress becomes persistent, long-overlooked symptoms become unseen. Milling tooth, tremors, misunderstandings, forgetfulness, over-eating, and alcoholism are simply a number of the signs that appear to be practices that are as durable as the situations that triggered most of them.

Stress indicators might help most of us measure the amount of stress. However, stress symptoms frequently overlap from a single level to another. Moreover, many symptoms of stress could be triggered by just physical diseases or mental disorders.

Spotting stress symptoms might help us inhibit anxiety and stress from mounting; from severe to persistent, this quickens us to get medical help if we require it, and saves us from struggling the debilitating implications of stress.

Chapter 4

Effects of Stress

The results of worry can significantly affect one's existence for either better or worse. The rush of adrenalin, released during severe stress, provides us with an escape if we want to retreat from the situation or a supplementary surge of power if we choose to stand and battle.

However, if we don't put-off stress by merely coping with life's situations, this accumulates until we possibly explode or collapse. The results of stress could cause particular disorders in both mind and body, furthermore, towards the rising of the human stress hormones: Adrenaline and Corticosterone. Accumulated stress could cause headaches, digestive problems, eating disorders, sleeping problems, exhaustion, and lower the amount of resistance to other ailments, just like the common cold and flu.

If we are deluged with some stressful circumstances, our

bodies usually do not take the time and energy needed to change, neither do our thoughts proffer decisions necessary to help us keep up with the pressure. That's episodic stress!

After a while, unrelieved stress like occasional stress can result in increased heart rate, respiration, and blood pressure, which puts unnecessary stress on organs like the heart and lungs.

Ultimately your body suffers in the combat; struggling to rescue it from your complications, you develop more significant complications like coronary disease, high blood circulation pressure, heart stroke, and additional health problems.

Long-term pressure becomes persistent stress. The pressure comes off traffic, underlying every feeling of hopelessness, continuous panic, depressive disorder, and in serious instances, severe mental aberration such as paranoia and delusions. And suicide is without a doubt the worst effect of stress.

Just like every individual's reactions vary, there is no limit concerning the amount of stress every folk can simply endure. Every individual is endowed with their own stress "thermometer." When the mercury plummets, we must have a well-planned strategy to manage anxiety so we can stay healthy as we ought to. Knowing and employing a handful of stress administration tips will make all the difference in the results.

Chapter 5

Stress Administration Tips

Not all anxiety is bad. Stress may bring change, helping us focus on what's essential and to conserve our lives. However, when stress accumulates, it could result in the opposites- and cause most of us to spin our tires, keep us from focusing, and trigger physical damage as well as premature death.

The first suggestion for dealing with stress will be to identify your stressors, i.e. what stresses you. The next phase is dealing with them.

Another Stress management hint based on several old and also some new adages can help you perform that.

Concentrate and take a deep breath and count from number 1 to Ten - Taking a deep breath provides the body with oxygen, which is usually very quick and will help you to relax. Furthermore, taking an instant to breathe can help you regain your composure, which generally overtime is the logical thing to do in a tense situation.

Take time to relax - Remember, rest is usually contrary to anxiety and stress.

Laugh - You'll feel better and livelier!

Take a brief walk - Take a glass of water. Do something that distracts you from the problem. Whenever you're ready to sort out the problem, most likely, it won't appear insurmountable.

Smell the Roses - "Things happen" and sometimes "bad things happen to good people." If we allow them to, tense occasions can build-up wall structures and prohibit us from savouring the excellent beauty of life.

Try - Frequently, most of us place the pleasantries of existence around the trunk burner, telling ourselves we don't have "have time" or can't "make out time" for them.

However, time might be the thing most of us do own. Even though we can't "own" the whole day that's a lot longer than daytime, we all start our day around the same timeframe, and have an element of energy to identify the stunning items within our daily life.

Sleep on it - Every gold coin has two sides. Every concern offers both positives and negatives. Make a list of them both, then, put the list away and also have a second look through it the following day. Sometimes "sleeping on" a predicament changes the minuses to pluses.

Every cloud has a silver lining. In the long run, rainfall makes plants grow! Bill Franklin discovered sound within bolt lightning. Uncover the good stuff inside your nerve-racking situation by listing the harmful surges and identifying what it would take to turn them into pleasant situations.

Know your limitations - Understanding yourself plus your restrictions may be the standard approach to controlling stress effectively.

Challenges sometimes makes it difficult to make proper decisions or in giving a "yes" or "no". Yet this decision is another little thing that maybe the "straw that breaks the camel's rear." It is alright to say "No," "I can't," or

"Later."

Quit blaming yourself - Occasionally, situations are uncontrollable, and it might not be your fault that things turned out the way they did. So learn to stop chiding yourself!

Be pro-active to discover serenity – Those that heavily depend on medicine or alcohol to help ease stress often end up needing help or seeing a therapist, whereas for the mainstays it might just be a prayer of tranquillity:

"God grant me the courage to simply accept the things I can't change; the composure to boost the things I can; as well as the ability to comprehend the difference."

If you'd like help, get help! Atlas can't carry the weight of the world on his neck forever! Whether you'll need support from your kids or partner in hauling household goods into the house; advice from a pal to solve a work-related issue; or specialized support to obtain the causes of and efficiently manage your stress. Getting the assistance you'll need is usually alone a substantial stress management suggestion!

Other Suggestions

- Sleep well at night.

- Eat healthy meals.

- Listen to your favourite music.

- Workout - Be part of a sport or any fun activity.

- Map out your time and energy and prioritize.

- Have someone you can talk to about your challenges, preferably a close pal. Don't bottle it all up.

- Get a massage therapy.

- Rest.

- Have a warm shower.

- Read a book or watch television.

Chapter 6

Managing School Stress

Remember that old proverb that asks "Is the cup half-empty or 50 percent total?" this adage asks about whether a glass which has 50 percent water and 50 percent air is half full or half empty. Obviously, no matter which way you decide to answer, the glass provides the same amount. Good, this technique as regards stress and peace will help you control either high school or university stress.

Everything you've got is undoubtedly one year ahead you, but it's instead a year filled up with achievement or a 12 month filled up with stress, based on your plan.

Among the functions of education, usually, is to solve problems, and using this method, get ready for the downsides of life after college. Learning how exactly to fair in managing school stress will certainly bring you a considerable victory in handling stress in your life.

The secret to high school and university stress is organization.

See college as your short-term business - You can't work in an office without materials; in the same similitude, make sure that your paper, pencils, pens, files, etc. are well-stocked. Personal suggestions on how best to reduce school stress:

· Keep your locker well-organized.

· If you'd need help with a subject, don't hesitate to find a teacher. Educators and professors can offer advice.

· Strategize and work out your plan - Time created for research ought to be strictly adhered to, unless an authentic crisis (open fire, overflow, and famine) gets in the way. If you need to rest after classes, you can rest but commit your time and effort to do research later at night. Remember that rest is contrary to stress and be sure to include both in your time-table.

- Particular Suggestion: Don't allow work build-up to screw up your weekend. Even though you decide to study anytime on Saturday or Sunday, make one of these days your "day off." You'll find that facing the new week is easier when you've experienced real-time to refresh!

- Prioritize - You will find books you'd need to read, and also you cannot read all at the same time. Pick them one at a time.

1. Concentrate on extended tasks or;

2. Proceed through a section (or several pages) forward.

Select a friendly subject matter - Whenever you're tasked with finding a subject matter, choose something associated with your passion, not necessarily what you think will impress the educator.

Apart from making assignments more pleasurable and

less demanding; good grades are gotten from great work, so do your best to get good results, and revel in everything you do.

Cramming is an excellent method to learning faster. It is necessary to be viewed occasionally; nevertheless, you might prevent physical pains and aches (stressors) and innovate blocks by taking a five-minute break after each hour of research.

Stop wasting time - Unless you have a reasonably thick meticulous exam schedule, classroom peanuts and educators' intelligence are bound to make you feel unpleasant. Discover just as much as you can in the areas of concentration in regards to the examination. Consider the advantage of any practice assessments.

Know the type of test - Multiple-choice examinations are often about truth, method, and data. Article assessments typically require you to have an understanding of them and perhaps get into details with a topic or two.

Ensure you get and organize all you will need a night before the exam. Stock your handbag or briefcase with whatever you think you'll need a treat, water, calculator, eyeglasses, etc.

Avoid taking meals before an exam - There won't be ample time or opportunity to take meals. Apart from making you fatigued, a filled tummy may also make you stressed and shaky.

Go for success - Whether you work hot or chilly, the region could be out of a safe zone. Wear mild clothing suitable for your skin and a proper sweater or coat you could shed in an unneeded event.

Chapter 7

Helping Kids Reduce Stress

Kids usually learn by examples; they do what they observe. The best way to teach your kid how exactly to control stress is usually to apply the content at Pressure Management Suggestions to work out how to successfully manage your stressors. More so, you can develop skills and child-oriented stress management methods to help your kids identify and manage their unique stressors.

Eat healthily - A sound body combats stress-induced disease better. Plan regular foods and treat times. Don't allow your kid to skip meals.

Strenuous exercise is a superb stress reliever - The same as adults, kids, want time and energy to relax. If your kids are tied to gambling, television, or a computer, make them get on their feet and initiate the use of active playthings like balls, strike handbags, and bikes. The time spent together with your children is an excellent way, to get them to start a conversation.

Be clear in establishing rules and firm with self-discipline. Children have a home in a "black and white" world. Blurry recommendations and inconsistencies are a lot more complicated with them than they might be for adults.

Mild physical touch is an excellent healer - Occasionally, a hug could be more significant than a thousand words. Yet another physical stress reliever could be a mild massage therapy from the child's throat and neck.

Be a great listener - Whenever your son or daughter really wants to discuss his/her complications, don't criticize. More so, everything isn't about giving good advice. Occasionally kids want to chat. Motivate them with open-ended questions like, "What happened exactly?" "How would you like to experience this?"

Teach your kids that everybody (including you) make mistakes. A fantastic start is admitting your errors to your children with an "I'm sorry" or "My mistake" when you goof-up. If the problem deserves attention, tell stories of stressful situations you experienced during childhood.

While you weren't successful in dealing with your challenges, you'll train your kids and tell them about it and even giggle at the mistakes together.

Finally, train your kids to engage in worry-relieving exercises and help them to discover stress-reducing games they could perform to reduce their anxiety.

Chapter 8

Stress-Relieving Online games

When stress mounts and frustration develops, it's a sure indication of stress. Playing a stress-relieving game can help you relax, and it's an effective way to get over the feeling of anxiety. The trick of stress-relieving video games will be to try types you can understand easily and enjoy. What you will do is show yourself you can be successful. Once you get yourself a few "wins" below your belt regularly, you'll begin to see the original issue from a new perspective.

Video games

From beating a floor hog to batting a rugby ball, you will find lots of flash video games on the internet, and also, most of them are fascinating to take pleasure from. The best way to bunch your anti-stress arsenal is usually to look for "Free Adobe flash Video games" or "Display Video games" and bookmark them has your favourite. You can also play the free (or paid) game on your mobile phone or tablet by installing the sport application on your device.

Offline Stress-relieving video games

If you're seated the whole day with a computer, occasionally, the very best break is to get up and leave. Below are few video games that are easy to play and excellent to help you to reduce stress:

Got a deck of cards? Play solitaire game the old-fashioned way! Using your deck, you might consider purchasing a publication of Solitaire video game. Many books are released explicitly for Solitaire players and offer numerous video games and game variants.

· Rubik's Dice - This is a suggestion: Anyone may match an individual side from the Rubik's dice.

· Slinky – Simply moving a slinky backward and forwards from an accessible point puts your focus on the toy and demands this for your trouble. So jump your slinky, have several deep breaths, and unwind!

· Punch tennis balls - Ok, they're not really a game;

however, they could be considered a fantastic pressure reliever, and they're sure a far better decision than striking a wall or throwing the medial side from the table when stress occurs! You will find cheap impact balls in toy departments, novelty shops, and most buck stores.

· Darts - Whether you're trying to concentrate on a graphic, the physical movement of tossing the darts alone might help lessen your stress. Dart tennis balls abide by a Velcro table. They'll not harm you or your neighbour - in the event that you miss!

Crossword Puzzle - Many crossword puzzle books likewise incorporate word-finding video games, mazes, and different additional pencil questions. Buy several that have questions that range between simple to hard and cope with them relating to your feeling plus your stress level!

Chapter 9

Stress Relieving Exercises

Although you may not consider exercise has been stress alleviating (if you've ever had a home training for any pressure test), sound health is a formidable tool to fight stress.

A complete workout program may not be easy to complete, yet several easy exercises can be carried out to assuage pressure and reduce stress. Even when your task is usually challenging, the activities are designed to help you relax and minimize stress.

Screw it up off - Yoga breathing turns up naturally, and it is generally overlooked, yet it's an excellent stress reducer. Breathe in a while, tucking in your tummy and inhale the air; it develops your bronchi plus your chest muscles. Breathe inward, count from one to four, and do this for two minutes, and then breathe out.

Take 2 to 4 deep breaths each day, and daily stressors could be "eliminated with all the blowing wind!"

Take a brief walk after lunchtime - A ten or fifteen-minute walk each day isn't only literally beneficial, yet shifts your concentration from the landscapes along your way, to the good-looking person in the hall or the timber inside a nearby park.

Press a lemon. P. T. Barnum stated, "When life hands you a "lemon," make lemonade!" Blending a citrus or rugby ball is a superb way to keep the fingernails and from gnawing at in the hands. Should you smash the fruits or the baseball, possibly get yourself a plastic ball or steadily move on to a more strenuous exercise to reduce your stress!

Progressive rest is especially needed when stress keeps you from finding a sound night sleep - Make sure every part of your body from your mind to your feet gets rest.

The very best feeling at that time ought to be serenity through your body; foot, ankles, quads, legs, thighs, etc. Up to your chest muscles, your neck, and finally, to your brain or down your hands (if you make everything easier before you're asleep!)

Dance - Join a fitness class, a Tai Chihuahua class, or join the music and dance class. Dance includes a two times advantage along with exercise. And music is an excellent stress reducer.

Chapter 10

What Makes Children Anxious Today?

Consider all the things that may trigger anxiousness in an average adult's day: Sound, digital activation from televisions, computers, cell phones, and other continuous information-emitting devices, targeted prospects, shuffling functions and responsibilities, actions, and family. For kids, who tend to be susceptible to sound and uproar, day-to-day stress triggers could be amplified, making the needed silence a lot more critical. Increasing college and after-school actions, the pressure to have success (whether it's from within or outside), family adjustments or issues, and a couple of elements that may bring about anxiety as well as the perfect formula for kid's stress.

Indicators of Stress in Kids

Often, kids, especially younger children, cannot wholly

express their emotions of anxiety and stress. The symptoms of stress in children may be quite delicate, such as abdominal pains and aches, headaches, or changes in behavior. You may see mood swings and sleep issues as well as difficulty focusing at school.

If there have been any changes in a child's existence like relocation or a new sibling, parents should carefully observe feasible indicators of the child's stress. While you cannot pinpoint a particular stress element, your kid might experience anxiety from something at school or several other factors that might be oblivious to you.

Monitor his/her behavior and moods, watching for just about any sign of problem. Inquire his/her instructor about how exactly he/she is doing in school and observe him/her, if he/she is interacting with family and friends.

Additionally, it worth talking to your kids about how they feel, although they might not have the ability to express it in "grown-up" language. Ask questions on what they might be worried about or factors that might be responsible for the edgy feeling. Generally, youngsters will not understand these words as anxiety or stress.

What parents should do about kids' stress

Make your children understand they have access to talk to you - Encourage your kids to talk to you about any complications they might be having, and to discuss their feelings freely and truthfully. Talking to somebody about their problem is one of the most crucial and effective ways humans can put-off stress.

Even if your kids have challenges in communicating what they are actually angry about, having you ask and initiating conversations can change things.

Be sure to listen to your kids before offering recommendations - As much as you could jump in and offer solutions, allow them to express their thoughts and feelings before making comments, or expressing your opinions.

Consider performing a task while you chat - Some kids maybe comfortable discussing their problems while performing a task with either of their parents. Choose an activity you both enjoy, like going for a walk, baking cookies, or playing baseball in the driveway right before asking your kids to talk about any challenge they could be having.

Research asserts that males are comfortable voicing their emotions if they are involved in an exercise while talking.

Get children to do several yoga breathing exercises - Encourage children to inhale "good" airflow and exhale "bad" atmosphere, and picture it being transported out of their bodies.

Do some Pilates poses together with your children - Basic yoga exercises position such as downward dog, cobra, and tree are excellent for kids. While you do this for some time, every day before college or at night right before going to bed, just a little peace with you can make a significant change in a child's day.

Try some quick stress-relief ideas for kids - These kinds range between fun activities you can enjoy with one another. Snuggling with a book, therapeutic massage, or playing a favorite game.

How to handle Anxiety in Children

It's unfortunate yet an accurate fact that anxiety and stress in children is, without a doubt, a common problem in today's fast-paced, high-tech, and activity-packed society. If your kid is usually experiencing anxiety and stress, try these simple yet effective solutions to support and her manage her fear of getting worried, and annoyed.

· Don't write off her emotions - Telling your kid not to be mindful of her anxieties might only help to make her feel like she's doing something wrong just by being stressed. Let her know it is alright to feel bad about something and encourage her to talk about her feelings and thoughts.

· Listen – You'd realize how comforting it is to have someone give you attention when something's bothering you. Do a similar thing for your kid. If they don't feel like talking, simply tell them you will always be there for them. You should be concerned about their actions and constantly remind them that you want and support them.

· Provide Comfort and Distraction - Make an effort to do something they love, like playing a favorite game or cuddling them in your lap and having you read with them.

· Take them Outdoors - Exercise can boost their sensation, thus get them moving. Sometimes it's merely a walk around, oxygen and exercise could just be what might lift their spirits and give them a fresh perspective to viewing things.

· Stick to routines - Balance any adjustments by adhering to their regular schedule. Try to stick to proper bedtime and meals when possible.

Sustain your son or daughter's health

Make sure he's eating right and getting a lot of rest. Getting inadequate rest or eating not too balanced meals over a period of time can contribute to your child's stress. If he feels good, he'll be well-equipped to straighten out whatever is bothering him.

· Avoid Overscheduling

Soccer, fighting techniques, football, music lessons, and other groups of extracurricular activities kids might take on are endless. So many activities can lead to anxiety and stress in children. Just like grown-ups require some rest after work, and on weekends, children likewise need some peace.

· Avoid upsetting news

If your kid views or listens to upsetting pictures or news about natural disasters, such as earthquakes or tsunamis or views disturbing reports of assault or terrorism on the news, educate your kid about what's happening. Reassure her that the people she loves and cares about aren't in danger.

Tell her that people who are victims of disasters or violence have gotten help from humanitarian or education groups, and discuss how she might help.

· Consider seeing a Counselor or Physician

In the case where there is an adjustment in the family such as a new baby, relocation, divorce, or the death of a loved one in the family causes your kid's anxiety and stress, talk to an expert such as your kid's college counselor, your pediatrician, or a children therapist. They can recommend methods on how to discuss death with kids, or support them through some other change in the family.

· Plan a Quiet Example

You can set the tone on how exactly anxiety and stress in adults and children are handled in your home. You can practically draw up suggestions on how to filter stress from your lives in today's high-tech, 24-hour-news-cycle world; nevertheless, you may have to take action on how precisely to handle your stress.

Switch off, play some soothing music, and try some comforting yoga postures and extra stress-relieving strategies. The better you're able to retain calmness and peace in your home, the unlikely it is that kid's anxiety and stress can be an issue in your home.

Chapter 11

Preventing Vacation Anxiety and Stress in Children.

The vacation season is a superb and memorable time; nevertheless, also an exceptionally busy one, and vacation anxiety and stress in children is one of the things you have to deal with. During vacations, several fun activities and events happen, both at homes and in school.

Even though this might be an essential activity the simple truth is that it tends to be hectic, meaning activities tend to be enjoyable, bedtimes extended, and routines interrupted. As a result of this, kids might inevitably experience some degree of vacation stress.

Become an example

The major way parents might help relieve anxiety in children during the holiday could be by attempting to keep them relaxed. Like in most situations, how parents manage a problem may set the tone for how their children will react. When you allow the holiday stress get to you, kids will know it, and a stressed kid is likely the least thing you would like to deal with during the holidays.

To lessen nervousness in kids during vacations, ensure to deal with your anxiety and stress.

· Setup conditions for behavior

Avoid taking your kid to places like the retail center or vacation gatherings when he's hungry or exhausted. It's hard for a grown-up to handle noise and lots of activities when they're not in the right mood; kids become hungry and exhausted frequently, and may throw tantrums; discuss essential behaviors and how to overcome holiday stress.

· Remember to stick to schedule

The holidays can disorganize schedules in the home, and this may come with its own stress. To lessen vacation stress for your kids, try to put habits on the right course once a gathering or party is finished. For instance, if a college vacation concert or a chapel gathering would take place before your kid goes to bed, try to adhere silently to informal actions the next day and ensure your kid goes to bed promptly.

· Watch what they eat

Avoid all the excess sugary vacation snacks that makes it impossible to eat regular foods, maybe it's easy for kids to take less balanced meals, but that could also contribute to vacation anxiety and stress in children. Try making healthy snacks, when you have to cook during vacation, ensure you reduce the amount of sweet treats eaten in the home, offer healthy snacks like popcorn or apple pieces with cheese products and crackers and limit cookies and candy to after-snack goodies.

· Get Your kid Moving

Oxygen and workout are necessary to improve mood and uplift the spirit in assuaging vacation anxiety and stress in children. Ensure you create time to get your kid outside to walk around and play.

· Prevent Overscheduling

The allure of the vacation might require the presence of family and friends. Try to limit your vacation celebrations and activities so you and your kids don't get too confused as regard the arrival of a large number of people. Many weekly occasions maybe beautiful, yet having an event every day can lead to vacation anxiety and stress in children.

Grown-ups prefer to help their parents, mainly because they get a lot of commendation of being accountable and helpful. When you have to work, ask your kids to assist you in looking for something in the shop (fun stocking for cousins, for instance). Giving your child a sense of responsibility will not only increase his/her self-pride; it'll distract her and help to prevent any holiday anxiety and stress.

· Have peaceful moments together

Having some tranquility with your child is usually more important than whatever you share during the Christmas season. Select a book and read a chapter or passage together, or design vacation pictures for grandpa and grandma.

A fantastic antidote for you to put-off vacation stress, as well as the puffed-up commercialism from the growing season, is by supporting others, whether it's by shoveling a senior neighbor's pavement or by merely wrapping presents for clingy kids in the town's chapel. Helping your child become charitable might help relieve her vacation anxiety and stress.

Chapter 12

Handling Anxiety and Stress in Kids

Signs of anxiety and stress in kids often start out as physical or behavioral changes. Kids react differently to stress with regards their age, personalities, and coping abilities that may trigger many parents to discover the underlying conditions, which may be responsible for their child's behavior.

Parents have to identify the symptoms of kid's stress and seek out the possible causes. Parents can generally help kids manage anxiety and stress; however, many kids will come with panic and would require the help of a specialist.

Signs of Stress in Kids

Children may not recognize their panic and stressful problems. This might require a set of physical and behavioral symptoms to emerge, and parents may be uncertain if the symptoms are that of stress or not.

Common indicators of anxiety and stress are:

- Behavioral or Emotional adjustments.

- Having problem concentrating.

Behavioral changes – this is usually moodiness, aggression, tantrum, or clinginess.

Signs to consider are;

- Been taken away from family or friends.

- Refusal to go to school.

- Having trouble at school.

Physical

- Reduced or increased hunger.

- Incessant abdominal pains or headaches.

- Bedwetting.

- Inability to sleep or constant nightmares.

Additional physical symptoms

It will help if you are able to discern whether these symptoms happen before or after some specific activities and whether you will see physical symptoms, such as pain, fevers, allergy, or diarrhea that could mean a medical problem.

Common Causes of Stress in Children

The building blocks of stress in kids could be something external, just like a problem at school, changes in the family, or disagreement with a friend. Some common causes of anxiety in children are:

- Significant Changes in the Family

Main life adjustments that may result in children's anxiety include divorce, a death in the family, relocation, or possibly the birth of a new sibling. These kinds of seismic adjustments can rock your child's world. Main life adjustments can shake your child's sense of security, leading to confusion and stress. For example, "a new cousin could make a kid vulnerable and envious."

- Parent Instability

Cash and work concerns, family turmoil, and parental disappointment can lead to a sense of powerlessness for children who may wish to support but don't possess the ability to do so.

- Monotony

Continuously engaging in an activity repeatedly can result in a whole lot of stress for kids who love varieties.

- Academic Pressure

Many kids become tensed about wanting to do well at school. Academic pressure is typical in kids who are scared of making mistakes or who are worried about not been productive at something.

- Recognition

For young children, this anxiety could be considered a

universal problem. Because they get older, and wants to be friends with kids who have high self-esteem and be like them, the pressure to fit in and be well-known could be distressing. Cliques and the feeling of not belonging can really make a child worried once he begins school.

Bullying is generally a significant concern for some kids, and may bring about physical damage.

Children who are bullied often feel ashamed, and they might choose not to tell their parents or instructors about the harassment.

Catastrophic events on the news

Info headlines and pictures talking about natural disasters, terrorism, and assault could be distressing for kids. When children see and hear about awful events, they could easily become worried that something terrible may happen to someone they like.

A Frightening Movie or a Book

Imaginary stories could also scare or stress kids. Children

usually experience frightening, violent, or upsetting moments from a show or movie. Some children are more delicate to please than others, and it's brilliant to know precisely what might upset your kid, limit violent media content, and abide by age-appropriate films, books, games, and additional press restrictions.

How to Support Your kid

You will see that your kid often responds to stress in a healthy way; they just require some help and assistance. You can help using the following techniques:

At Home

- Make your home a calm, safe, and sound place to relax.

- Create a relaxed atmosphere and come up with programs. Family member's meals or game evenings can prevent panic and lessen stress and make sure they are involved.

- Monitor your kid's TV shows, games, and books.

- Provide your kid with prior notice on any anticipated adjustments which would happen shortly. For example, if you will be taking a new job in a new town, what this means to them is that they are moving into a new school, having new friends, and a new home.

- Involve your kid in social activities and sports, wherever they can easily achieve success.

- Adopt healthy behaviors, the type that helps to control your stress in healthy ways. Kids often imitate their parents' actions.

- Offer affection and encouragement.

- Make use of positive encouragement and means of self-discipline that promote healthy self-esteem.

- Figure out how to relate with your kids and never having to end up being critical.

- Offer to assist your kid and proffer solutions to comprehending and solving the problems that irritate them.

- Look out for new signals and actions of conflicting

stress.

Seek help from the healthcare practitioner, counselor, or therapist if the signs of stress do not reduce or if your kid becomes more withdrawn, consumed with stress, or highly unsatisfied. Complications in college or in interacting with friends or family can be another cause for concern.

Panic is an all-too-common problem faced by kids today. Concerning a child's anxiousness, young children might not have the capability to grasp or express their emotions.

Older children might understand what's disturbing them, although that's hardly any assurance that they'll discuss it with their father or mother. Being aware of changes in your kid's behavior will undoubtedly let you notice complications before they affect your kid.

Chapter 13

Stress Management Ideas

People who work on out how to cope with stress and business live a happier, healthier life; below are a few ideas to help you put away stress.

- Maintain a proper attitude.

- Accept there are circumstances you can't control.

- Be assertive rather than being aggressive.

- Be firm with your feelings, opinions, or values instead of becoming furious, defensive, or aggressive.

- Go outdoor and practice relaxation methods; try yoga, Pilates, or tai-chi solely to relieve stress.

- Exercise frequently. Your body will be better equipped to combat stress if it is fit.

- Eat balanced meals.

- Figure out how to manage your time and energy

effectively.

-   Know your limits and learn to avoid activities that could result in extreme stress.

-   Create time for interests, passions, and relaxation.

-   Get enough rest. Your body needs time to revive from nerve-racking occasions.

-   Avoid depending on alcohol, drugs, or compulsive behaviors to reduce anxiety and stress.

-   Seek out friendly support. Spend the time with those you like.

-   Consult psychiatrists or other mental doctors who have been trained to manage stress or bio-feedback methods to learn healthy approaches of dealing with your stress.

Breathing Approaches to Stress Relief

-      Take a breath in, and then breathe out. You may notice a remarkable difference in how you feel already. Your breathing is a healthy method to significantly ease stress. Several simple respiration exercises will make a huge difference if you can be consistent with them.

Before starting, have the following tips in mind:

ü   Choose where to execute your breathing exercise . Maybe it's on your bed, on your living-room floor, or a chair. This might make you more comfortable, wear comfortable clothes and make an effort to do the exercise several times a day.

ü   Engage in lots of yoga breathing exercises, which takes a couple of minutes. When you have more time you can do them for 10 minutes or more to get continuous benefits.

ü   Meditation: Lots of people take short, superficial breaths. You might have experienced stress and have your energy zapped but with this technique, you may learn how to take bigger breaths, into your stomach.

ü   Get comfortable - You can lie on your bed or floor with a cushion under your head and legs, or you might sit in a chair together with your neck, head, and throat backed against the seat, and breathe through your nose.

ü   Fill your stomach with air.

ü   Inhale through your nose.

ü   Place one hand on your stomach.

ü   Place the other hand on your upper body.

ü   As you draw in breath, your tummy rises;

ü   And as you exhale, it reduces.

Breathing Focus

When you do yoga breathing exercise, create a mental picture in your mind to help you feel better.

ü   Close your eyes if they are open.

ü   Take several deep big breaths.

ü   Breathe – And as you do that, imagine that your surrounding is filled peace and tranquility. Try to feel the peace in your body.

ü   Breathe out – while you do that, imagine your stress leaving the environment along with what you're exhaling.

ü   Now coin a phrase or expression to go with your breathing.

ü   As you breathe say: "I breathe in peace and tranquility."

ü   As you breathe out say:, "I breathe out stress and pressure."

ü   Continue for ten to twenty minutes.

With this workout, you'll measure how long you breathe-in and out. After a while, your breathing span is likely to increase.

ü   Sit comfortably on the floor or on a chair.

ü   Breathe through your nose; and count from one to five.

ü   Gently expel your breathe through your nose after counting from one to five.

ü   Exercise often.

Once you become comfortable with holding in breaths for 5 minutes, try keeping your breathe in for several more minutes, you can try to hold it in for ten minutes.

Intensify muscle tissue relaxation

In this technique, you produce a muscle tissue when you breathe. Intensifying muscle tissue relaxation might help you relax physically and psychologically.

ü   Lie comfortably on the floor.

ü   Take several deep breaths to unwind.

ü   Breathe in; tense the muscles of your toes.

ü   Take in air. Launch the strain inside your foot.

ü   Breathe in. Tense your quads.

ü   Exhale the air. Dissolve the tension in your calves.

This helps to make every part of the body function properly; your lower limbs, stomach, chest muscles, fingers, hands, shoulders, and throat.

Modified Lion's Breath

ü   While you exercise, imagine you're a lion. Allow yourself to breathe out through the mouth.

ü   Sit comfortably on the floor or on a chair.

ü   Inhale through your nose and draw in air into your tummy.

ü   Open the jaws as large as you can. Breathe in and out with an "Ahh."

ü   Do it frequently.

Techniques for dealing with stress are determined by the complexities in your life. As effortless as it seems, many people are not conscious of what gives them anxiety. What stresses someone out might be another's inspiration.

Likewise, few people realize their particular thoughts, emotions, and manners attributes to what stresses them. Most of us are in charge of how we interpret situations in our lives. We are responsible for habits such as procrastination, unfinished business, and negligence towards our businesses, which leads to deadline, not being prudent with our expenses and failure to carry out important jobs which subsequently triggers stress.

Consequently, the first stage is to identify the stressors and stress in your life and the methods to be employed in overcoming them.

·   Simplify your lifestyle - If you are wearing yourself out by exercising too much, start reducing some of your unsuccessful, yet frustrating and energy-draining actions. No-one is capable of doing everything.

Similarly, it is crucial to learn how to say NO! Delegate and redistribute responsibilities when you have to, don't try to do everything. Get someone to do your cleaning for you, maybe once in a week. Hire a babysitter to sit the children after school, you don't have to do everything yourself.

Five suggestions for healthy living

· Reduce the tendency of being stressed by eating well, exercising frequently, and getting enough sleep – Most times, whenever we are hungry or exhausted, we become pressured and grumpy. Not getting the proper diet the body requires causes both mental and physical stress.

Regular physical exercises don't produce anxiety and stress; it rather generates endurance and helps you to cope better with pressure. Most people take for granted the need to be physically fit in order to combat stress and anxiety.

Advantages of Routine workouts

· Accept that there are things you can't change - As

everyone knows, there are so many things in life that are beyond control, e.g. the death of a loved one, loss of job, disease etc.

As hard as it might be to consent that certain things in life are beyond control and inevitable, it'd be better to understand that certain situations can't just be controlled. Also, we can choose how we react to these uncontrollable situations in the following ways:

·   Talking about what you're going through to a pal or therapist (recovery).

·   Keeping a diary to record thoughts and emotions (cathartic).

·   Discover new ways to develop; and learn from it (active).

·   Develop strength (building internal resistance).

There are many causes of unavoidable stress, such as a job interview, taking an exam, having to make a presentation, a disagreement with someone, and similar situations.

In many cases, it will be beneficial to learn how to remain as calm as possible. Take yoga breathing exercises, (rehearse the techniques), and plan yourself beforehand, and watch the stress ease off your body.

Managing stress in healthy ways

Are you dealing with stress with the right technique or not? If you're managing stress in a delicate way, you are compounding the problem. Delicate ways of managing stress include; taking alcohol, using drugs, taking tobacco, excessive addiction to TV. Stress management techniques help to eliminate your worries, and avoid problems generally.

If you are stressed, and you are still managing your stress using harmful techniques, you are only compounding the strain.

Everyone has unique responses to stress and how they choose to deal with it. The trick will be to discover what works for you.

Study explains that stress reducers determine how much you can rest physically and mentally. The technique works and does not require a particular position or place. For instance, in case you are trapped with visitors, or you're having difficulty drifting off to sleep, here's how to help yourself:

ü   Sit back comfortably. Close your eyes and take it easy with your muscle tissue.

ü   Breathe in deeply - to ensure you're taking deep breaths, place one of your hands on your stomach and the other on your upper body.

ü   Inhale through your nose, when you do so you would feel your abdomen (and not your chest muscles) rise.

ü   Gradually exhale, and focus on your breathing.

ü   If thoughts begin to interfere, avoid dwelling on any of them. Allow them to fade to the background and refocus on your breathing.

ü   You can choose to exercise if you feel stressed. Enduring it regularly for approximately 10 to 20 minutes each day can give you a relaxed mind, that could help you go through typical stressful conditions.

Healthier Solutions to managing stress:

· Meditation, yoga exercises, or biofeedback techniques are examples of mind influx therapy.

· Exercise by taking a walk, weight lifting, or running.

· Spend time at the beach, driving, or within a new neighborhood.

· Visit a close friend.

· Have a hot perfumed bath,

· Get a massage.

· Play soothing music.

· Watch a comedy movie - this helps to relieve pressure.

Harmful ways of dealing with stress:

· Extreme drinking.

- Using drugs or pills to unwind.

- Sleeping too much.

- Becoming addicted to TV.

- Withdrawing from interpersonal activities.

Consequences of enduring Stress:

- Negatively changes your body and mind chemistry (stress hormones and cortisol).

- Weakens your immune system.

- Cardiovascular disease, hyper stress, heart attack, and stroke.

- Depressive disorder of anxiety and stress.

- Ulcer and stomach pain.

- Pores, skin problem and thinning hair.

- Headaches and migraines.

- Sexual disorder.

Everyone knows that life can be stressful, occasionally it's preventable and other times it's not; nevertheless, if we firmly consider how we can manage stress and apply effective techniques to dealing with it, stress could be a functional part of everyday life.

Acknowledgements

The Glory of this book success goes to God Almighty and my beautiful Family, Fans, Readers & well-wishers, Customers, and Friends for their endless support and encouragement.

CPSIA information can be obtained
at www.ICGtesting.com
Printed in the USA
BVHW042333180221
600507BV00014B/1500